Weighed Down

Unlearning the Lies Sold to Us
About Our Bodies

**Mary Pearson,
Brigitte Botten & Nelly Rose**

First published in Far North Queensland, 2024 by Bowerbird Publishing

ISBN 978-0-6486041-4-3 (print)
ISBN 978-0-6486041-5-0 (ebook)

Weighed Down:
Unlearning the Lies Sold to Us About Our Bodies
By Mary Pearson,
Brigitte Botten & Nelly Rose

First edition: 2024

Edited by: Crystal Leonardi
Cover Concept & Design by: Mary Pearson & Crystal Leonardi
Interior Design by: Crystal Leonardi

Distributed by Bowerbird Publishing
Available in National Library of Australia

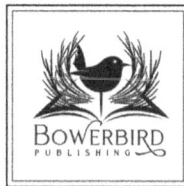

Crystal Leonardi, Bowerbird Publishing
Julatten, Queensland, Australia
www.crystalleonardi.com

To Veronica, for being alive at the same time as me.

Foreword

I met Mary Pearson at a professional development training course in Brisbane. Our anxious eyes met when asked to group with other participants for the experiential exercises. On the second day of the course, we had lunch and discussed the overlap of our professional and personal lives. Her passion for her career and the community she works with was evident. Still, there was also a sense of fun and silliness about her, a quality I share.

Over the last 15 years, my work has been primarily in bariatrics and eating disorders as a private practice clinician and presenter of educational courses for health professionals. I was intrigued when Mary mentioned her book, and I asked her if I could read the manuscript once it was completed. I admire Mary, Brigitte, and Nelly for the tenacity, vulnerability and truth contained within these pages. Absorbing the words and experiences of the authors may open people's minds to the possibility of changing their opinions about themselves and others.

We like to believe that societal attitudes have evolved in recent years. The media hashtags for #bodypositivity, #loveyourbody and #anti-diet are everywhere. However, these positive campaigns still exist alongside hashtags like #cleaneating, #superfoods, #detox, and #fasting. The fact that this book exists, and you are reading it, proves that we have yet to reach the point of this being a conversation we don't need to have.

Fatphobia drives our societal weight loss ambitions, and will always exist until it becomes unprofitable. It's Fatphobia that causes everyone to hate their bodies, regardless of size. Fatphobia does not cause fatness or thinness; it causes shame and self-hatred and supports a multibillion-dollar industry that is only too happy to sell you a 'solution'.

I have done much personal work on my body challenges over the years. I have a history of childhood trauma that led to panic attacks and an undiagnosed eating disorder for many years. When I became a therapist, it felt natural to try and help others escape from the thoughts and beliefs that had previously been influencing my behaviour.

I want to share a segment of my speech at an International Women's Day event a few years ago. I started by putting my hand in the air and asking the 300-plus women gathered to raise their hands if they had the perfect body. Everyone looked very confused, and there was nervous laughter, but no one raised their hand. I waited for a while. Then I said, "Oh... it's just me then?" More nervous laughter ensued, and perplexed expressions filled the crowd as they looked at my very average, other side of fifty body.

I explained that I did have the perfect body. I would have a different body if I were an athlete, a dancer, or a model. However, for me and the life that I live, it's perfect. My body has legs that are strong enough to carry me up a mountain in Nepal; those legs have allowed me to dance at parties and explore cities like London, Paris, Bangkok and Singapore. My body has eyes that allow me to escape into a fantasy world by reading a book or enjoying the beauty of a piece of art or architecture. My body has ears that enable me to listen carefully to the people I help each day and also enable me to relax by listening to music or hearing the words 'I love you.' My body has a brain that has allowed me to retain knowledge, solve problems, and experience love. My body has made two other human beings, an absolute miracle of nature. How did it know how to do that? My body has scars, stretch marks and wrinkles, but they are minor blemishes on something otherwise magnificent. My body has been doing miraculous things for over 55 years, and it's the perfect body for me.

I then asked the group to reconsider their thoughts about their body and what it does daily, and I ask you now to do the same. Put your hand up if you have the perfect body.

I'd like to finish with a quote I love. This is for anyone who criticises themselves, punishes their body, or believes they are insufficient.

"For some reason, we are convinced that if we criticise ourselves, the criticism will lead to change. If we are harsh, we believe we will end up being kind. If we shame ourselves, we believe we end up loving ourselves. It has never been true, not for a moment, that shame leads to love. Only love leads to love."

Geneen Roth.

Kyla Holley

Director and Therapist

The Australian Centre for Eating Behaviour

This is my body
And I live in it
It's thirty-one and six months old
It's changed a lot since it was new
It's done stuff it wasn't built to do
I often try to fill it up with wine
And the weirdest thing about it is
I spend so much time hating it
But it never says a bad word about me
This is my body
And it's fine
It's where I spend the vast majority of my time
It's not perfect, but it's mine.

-Tim Minchin

Contents

Author's Note

I am absolutely stoked that you picked up this book. What prompted you to do it? Can you relate to the feeling of being weighed down by the pressures of not looking and feeling good enough?

I will be completely transparent and tell you precisely what motivated me to start writing this book with my co-authors. I have listened to a myriad of people talk about how they are not pretty enough, thin enough, fit enough or curvy enough. They just can't seem to achieve this apparently simple goal of being enough, of looking the complete opposite to how they are.

Not believing your body is good enough looks like many things to me as a social worker. It looks like a 22-year-old woman caring for her sick parents daily instead of attending university, constantly feeding herself last at mealtimes. Her body screams for food because she is not eating throughout the day. Having no time to exercise or to treat her back issues and then the one time a year she can go into the city to socialise and get all dressed up, she chooses the grey and baggy long-sleeve top she doesn't like over the more revealing bright red top because her mother says big girls should cover up their skin. She then becomes that quiet girl in the corner, with low self-esteem and a low voice, surprised when someone pays attention to her and convinced that if they do, it is out of pity.

It looks like an 11-year-old trans girl who had changed schools three times already. She was bullied for growing her hair out and isolated herself as a way to cope with her arguing parents, disagreeing on the best way to handle her. She sneaks off to the bathroom to throw up two out of three meals a day because she believes that if she can be skinny enough, she will look as pretty as the other girls at school, and maybe a boy will like her.

It looks like a man who goes to the gym six days a week to become as big and robust as possible because, for the first twenty years of his life, he was skinny and told that he needed to eat more than the three meals a day he was already eating.

It looks like an eighteen-year-old student living with anxiety and depression, who used to starve themself because restricting what went into their body was the only sense of control they had in life. It took being in the hospital on a drip, surrounded by nurses to realise that if they didn't ask for help soon, they could die.

It's a confronting start to a book, I know. But that's the reality of the situation. I hope this book will help answer some questions you may have about our relationships with food, our bodies and ourselves. I use the word 'relationship' because our lives thrive on our connections, our love for something, someone, somewhere. Without relationships, life would be empty. Our relationships with our bodies should be of the utmost importance. After all, we've got them for life.

This leads me to answer the question of why reading this book is worth your attention. I want this book to spark a thought, provoke a conversation, or motivate you to ask a question that will lead you or someone you care about towards a more peaceful relationship with body and self. Quite grandiose, isn't it? Trying to influence the course of someone's life choices with words, but there are only so many other ways to go about it.

Through my work as a social worker, I have met many people during or soon after they experience a harrowing event. By developing a safe and respectful rapport, I can create space for people to speak as truthfully and as unfiltered as possible about their relationship with themselves and the world around them. Sometimes, I hear them say the cruellest things about themselves, and I want to tell them that I disagree with them. But that wouldn't help. So, I listen. That's one of the first skills social workers are trained in; active listening.

Through this support, I arm people with knowledge and strategies they can use to make more informed and empowered choices. But after years of supporting people during or immediately after painful events, there comes a time in many social workers' lives when they want to do more. That is why so many of us become early prevention workers, group facilitators, or writers. I want my life's work to help people who are suffering from thoughts of hatred for their bodies or struggling with behaviour that decreases their self-worth and increases their self-punishment.

This small collection of stories and research sits somewhere between a self-help book and an amateur journal article and, therefore, doesn't quite belong anywhere. Something I can relate to. I aim to share contemporary professional and personal insights on body image, mental health, food and fitness to a population fed lies and false promises by industries that don't care about the individual. My goal is to help every reader recognise that they are not alone and can make more informed choices.

The stories shared with you here are profound and honest.

Sometimes honesty can be embarrassing, like admitting that weight loss isn't about health but vanity. Humans are vain; we just are. It's in our biology to strive to look at what our tribe tells us is attractive so that we can feel accepted, safe and desired. We often apologise for it or try to hide the lengths we go for it. It is easy to be judged for going to extreme measures to change our bodies in the pursuit of beauty, but if we tell people, it is in the quest for health, how often are we questioned? Can we call out the wolf of pain under the sheep's clothing of health? Or better yet, can there be a reality where self-acceptance can exist alongside human vanity?

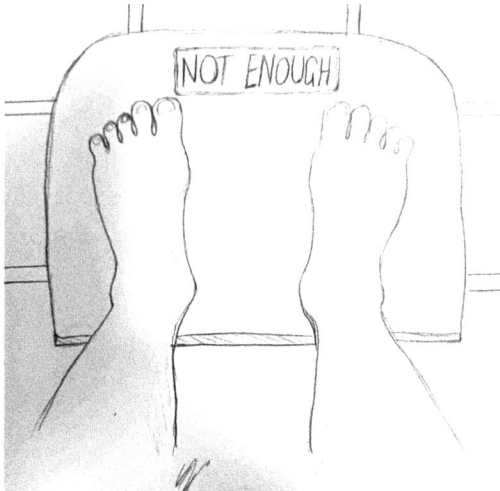

Sketch by Pearson, Dec. 2023.

Introduction:
There's no Such Thing as Bad Food

"As beauty standards shift through generations and cultures, we now hide our vanity behind the undisputable pursuit of health."

Mary Pearson

I sneakily write the first chapter of this book while at my work desk on a typically humid summer afternoon in Townsville, Queensland. Staring out my office window, I see the deep green edges of Mount Stuart. It's been raining a lot lately but typically; the scenery is mostly dry and dusty in Townsville so seeing green makes me happy. Unfortunately, my view is obstructed by a striking red and yellow McDonald's sign. The reminder of capitalism and consumerism has motivated me to write a note in my diary reminding myself to go for a waterfall walk this weekend to escape it all for a moment.

Instead of addressing the neglected pile of reporting, I take notice of comments made by the women in the office throughout the day. Come to think of it, what they say about themselves and others isn't new, I'm just paying more attention to them now.

"You look good. Have you lost weight?" I hear one woman attempt to compliment another in the photocopy room.

"No, it might just be that I am wearing black today. I always look thinner in black. But I am exercising daily to lose weight before my daughter's wedding", the other replies.

Two hours later, "Oh, you're so bad. Thank you, but I'm trying to be good." I hear another say while being offered a Tim Tam to go with her coffee.

Good and Bad. No matter how many posts I read or videos I watch stating the opposite, we still believe that losing weight is good and gaining weight is bad. Unless a doctor tells you that you must do one of them, "or else…", this is the status quo we follow. Even more preposterous than that, we continue to adhere to the rule that some foods are all good while others are all bad, which isn't true at all.

Co-author Brigitte Botten explains that a stomach doesn't know you have eaten a Tim Tam. It doesn't say, Oh no, it's another bad Tim Tam! It just registers that it now has new sugars, carbohydrates and sodium, which must be put to work or stored. The same goes for an apple. Your body doesn't know it's an apple, but it knows it has a boost of new sugars, carbohydrates, fibre, sodium and potassium. All foods serve a purpose, and the philosophical ideas of good and bad that we allocate to food are inaccurate.

Co-author Nelly Rose pointed me toward psychologist Glenn Mackintosh, who in his publications agrees that "food is not good and not bad, not right and not wrong, it's off the scale for moral judgement. There are no angel wings on your kale."

Looking at it more closely, I see that we easily allow our relationship with food to dictate our opinion of ourselves. "I'm trying to be good", we say, as if eating a Tim Tam can make you a bad person. Often underestimating the power of language, we allow negative self-talk to impact our mental health and how we truly think about ourselves.

Any good therapist will know the principal teachings of cognitive behaviour therapy, or CBT, which examines how our thoughts influence our feelings and behaviour, which, in a full circle, influences our thoughts. This tells us that if we say eating something is bad and restrict ourselves from eating it, we will believe we are good. Detrimentally, if we eat what we tell ourselves is bad, we will believe we are bad. It is a powerful personalised brainwashing we conduct upon ourselves. It's often a lot deeper than simply saying no to a Tim Tam.

1

Mary

All three authors in this book share insightful professional and personal experiences with the topic at hand. Depending on who is telling the story, you will notice different writing styles. Most of the time, however, it will be me.

Yes, I did not-so-subtly mention earlier that I, the lead author, am the social worker of the group. I have wanted to write about this issue for a long time as it confronts me regularly in my work. I'm overjoyed that Brigitte and Nelly have also shared their knowledge and experiences so that we can create a holistic and relatable resource. But before you get to know them properly, I'll humbly share my prequel to putting pen to paper or fingers to keyboard.

I had an epiphany at twenty-seven when, looking in the mirror, I found myself dissatisfied with my appearance and level of 'beauty.' This made me furious with myself because I was supposed to be 'body-positive.' I contemplated this conflict long and hard. I called friends about it, watched countless YouTube videos, read psychology articles, and interviewed people. What I learned was that the topic of body image and self-worth has been done to death. Yet, it needs to be re-learned a quadrillion times because humans, myself included, tend to repeat mistakes, especially when it comes to body image and self-worth.

I have always pursued an academic life. I love writing stories, speaking in front of crowds, having stimulating debates. In my ten years as a social worker, I have been able to embrace all of these interests and more. Throughout this time, I have also noticed that when it comes to being underestimated intellectually, I strive to prove my doubters wrong. But when it comes to my physical appearance, I measure my self-worth on other people's judgement and level of satisfaction.

I first started noticing my imperfections during the typical puberty years. I always labelled myself as 'over-weight', which translated to, "This is the thing about me that is bad". Now I hear similar stories from others: my clients, colleagues, family and friends, and I realise that we all look back on photos of ourselves when we were younger and say how beautiful we were. "I can't believe I thought I was fat", they would say.

I can recall only experiencing intense physical pain a few times in life:

• falling off a horse,

• waking up from anaesthesia after an operation,

• self-inflicted alcohol poisoning,

• humiliating food poisoning.

The worst of them all was the typical aftermath of a tonsillectomy. I was around fifteen when I had the operation. The pain in my throat felt like burning metal; the smell of rotting flesh was maddening, and it lasted for over a week, which felt like an eternity at the time. Swallowing my own saliva was agonising, and it made me cry every attempt. I could eat about three tablespoons of food daily, but it came with many more tears. I remember it being incredibly horrible for my mum. I expect it is torture for most parents to watch their child in pain. The doctor told me not to speak, as that would make the pain worse. So, I lay in my bed for days, trying to force myself to sleep the time away and remind myself it would be over soon.

After a week, the pain eased. It was still difficult to speak, but I made a croaky sound occasionally despite being reminded not to. My mum took me to a surf shop down the main street of our small town to buy me a new outfit to cheer me up. It was summer so I chose a T-shirt and floral swimming shorts. They fit perfectly.

While waiting for my mum outside the shop, I saw a school friend's mum as she was on her way to work at the chemist. She stopped to talk to me. She beamed at me and said, "You have lost a lot of weight. You look so good".

After she left, I looked at my reflection in the shop window. It did look like I had lost weight. But in my opinion, I didn't look that much different. I just looked like me. On the way home, I thought about what my friend's mum said and felt annoyed. I told myself she had good intentions, so why was it bothering me? I realised it was because I had not tried to lose weight. I was sick. I had been starving for a week. I had been in pain and was casually complimented for looking good. It was the first time I was confronted with the idea that I could impose self-inflicted starvation to look thinner. Thankfully, the idea did not stick.

As soon as the pain of the tonsillectomy had gone, I ate as much as possible for several days. I missed food, and food missed me. A few weeks later, I tried putting on the new outfit my mum bought me to go to the river with my friends. I put the shirt on effortlessly; then, I tried to pull the shorts on. They stretched over my thighs with a lot of effort, but it was to no avail, as the buttons could barely reach each other and, though I didn't realise it at the time, they were never going to again. I took the shorts off, folded them and put them at the back of my drawer. I put on some old baggy shorts and went to the river.

Years passed, and I was finally pursuing my academic career at university. I found that I did not take to the dangerously alluring vice of drugs like many of my peers. I did participate wholeheartedly in the culture of drinking and clubbing on the weekends. However, after dry-reaching a couple of times over a filthy toilet, I developed a habit of leaving the clubs early and returning to the safety and comfort of my bed in my share house.

To get me through my studies, I turned to the less talked about but much more accessible vice of comfort eating. It worked. When I ate four donuts in two minutes, the stress went away. Filling every gap in my mouth with the soft, sweet dough would trigger a long exhale through my nose. But the stress kept coming back. I didn't see this as a problem, so I didn't tell anyone about it. It wouldn't be for another decade that I would learn other ways to deal with stress. Sure, I still comfort eat, just not as much. And if I'm eating a donut, it's because I wanted it not out of habit.

Everyone has had issues with their relationship with food and how their bodies look at one point in their life. I believe this because I have never met anyone who has said they are delighted with every detail of how they look. Even if they were a sparkly unicorn, they would probably still think their horn could be slimmer.

All these memories of how I viewed myself came flooding back to me the more I met people with body dissatisfaction, body dysmorphia, or disordered eating. I reached out to my good friends Nelly and Brigitte to help me continue with this book because when they shared their stories with me, I was moved and challenged to evolve my way of thinking.

Nelly was a personal trainer and amateur pole dancer. She then became an empowered entertainer through erotic dancing (stripping) and competitive pole dancing. Nelly has always had a flair for rhetoric, and her contribution to this book is no exception.

Brigitte was a nutritionist who used to work in the weight loss industry. She eventually changed her career path and became an intuitive eating nutritionist and health coach, which has impressively resulted in her own business. These women have seen the realities of the fitness and weight loss industries firsthand.

2

Brigitte

My relationship with food and my body became very prominent during my teen years, like most females. In year nine, I first started to learn about food and nutrition and how they affect the body. Food and nutrition are so much more than the classic quotes. We have all heard, "You are what you eat", "Calories in, calories out", and "Junk food is bad", to name a few. My fifteen-year-old self was none the wiser, so I quickly adapted to this simple yet misguided way of understanding food and nutrition. I'd tell myself to eat clean, exercise regularly and stay thin. Notice I didn't say stay healthy? Well, that's because society has conditioned us to think that thin is healthy, happy and attractive and unhealthy is fat, unattractive and unloved. But to what extent are we striving for thinness? Well, it impacted my relationship with food and body for many years.

I grew up in a very large and low-income family with neglectful parents, leaving little room for nutrition and adequate food. When we could afford food, my siblings and I would attack the grocery bags before somebody unpacked them and put them away in the kitchen. My eating habits from childhood could be described as a feast or famine. I would either be so uncomfortable from eating way past fullness or intensely hungry that I found it hard to concentrate. There was no in-between.

After I finished high school, I travelled and worked in the UK and Europe. I had little money for food, and the eating habits that I learned at home did not serve me well. I tried intentional dieting for the first time, with the motivation to lose weight, as society had well ingrained the message that thinner was best. Before I returned home, I had this self-driven desire to lose more weight so that everyone could see this achievement. It led me to extreme dieting measures, and even though I was severely underweight (to the point where I no longer had regular menstrual cycles) it was never enough. I thought achieving a perfect body would equate to achieving love, happiness and confidence. I guess that's what society's message had imbedded into me.

No matter how 'good' I ate, it was never enough and the number on the scale was never low enough. Instead, I felt very depressed with low self-worth and low energy. This was the start of my struggle with a binge eating disorder and body dysmorphia. I became so obsessed with food; it was all I could think about. I was constantly focused on when, what, and how much food I would eat.

When we try to shrink our bodies by intentionally eating less, food becomes an obsession. This obsession is our body's way of ensuring we eat adequately and don't starve, ramping up hunger hormones in response to restriction. The hunger hormone Ghrelin stays elevated when you're undernourished or eat less, even after eating an average meal.

Being trapped in a pattern of restricting and binging is known as the diet pendulum, swinging back and forth between two opposite extremes. It is both mentally and physically exhausting. In my younger years, when I got too hungry, I would binge eat. After I binged, I would feel shame, guilt, self-disgust and uncomfortable in my body, telling myself that I would do better tomorrow, eat less, exercise more, and have more self-control. So, the vicious restrict/binge pendulum continued to swing.

There is a misconception that after we overeat or binge eat, we need to have more discipline and restrict food even more. However, to reduce binge eating and leave the restrict/binge pendulum, the body needs regular meals. A lack of willpower does not fuel this pendulum. Binge eating is a typical outcome of restriction.

After returning home from my travels, I enrolled in a university course for a Bachelor of Health Science and Food and Nutrition. It was not the best pathway to go down whilst I was already struggling with an eating disorder. Learning more in-depth details about food and nutrition only perpetuated my ingrained belief that 'clean eating' is good and 'junk food' is bad. This kind of black-and-white thinking fosters the belief that we should only be eating one way and anything else is deemed unhealthy, or better yet, the message that is quite notable, "Avoid certain 'junk foods' or you will gain weight."

I got to a point however, where I was so tired of spending my time, money and energy on this unhealthy, limiting and restrictive way of feeling, that I slowly started cultivating a healthier relationship with food and my body. I focused on learning intuitive nourishment and ditched the many diet rules to rebuild a healthier body image and begin respecting my body.

In the beginning, when I reverted to old habits, I felt guilty. Guilt should have no place in your eating experience as it plays a far more damning role in your overall health than the actual food you eat. Food rules are not helpful in a healthy relationship with food and will often get broken in due time, as we are not robots. Our bodies will override any rules and send craving messages to our brains so we allow ourselves to eat what we were avoiding in the first place.

Finally, when I removed rules and labels around my eating, I felt invigorated. I slowly re-introduced foods I had limited or restricted for so long. I took the time to figure out what satisfied and nourished me, allowing me to be more attuned to my body's hunger and fullness signals. As I slowly let go of the dieting shackles, I noticed that I was binging less and less. I experienced decreased preoccupation with food, reduced food judgements and started to eat to comfortable fullness.

My dieting history and disordered eating habits were driven by this firm, deeply imbedded belief from society's message to be slim and beautiful. Body image has nothing to do with what we look like and everything to do with how we think and feel about our bodies.

I focused my energy on body acceptance when working on rebuilding a healthy body image. Body acceptance doesn't mean loving your body all the time. That's just unrealistic, especially at the start. It does not focus on the body's appearance; instead, it focuses on respecting and caring for your body, acknowledging the feelings you have with your body, good or bad, and working through these feelings.

It is achievable to rebuild a healthy body image and feel good about our shape or size. When we feel good about ourselves, we are more likely to have a healthier relationship with food and our bodies.

Every individual is different, but everyone can have this conversation with themself. Ask yourself what you want beyond the image to feel more empowered and in control of your life. To me, that feels much better than someone else planning my meals and stuffing them full of turmeric. I hate turmeric.

3

Brigitte: Fatphobia

"Low self-esteem is a goldmine and fatphobia is the pickaxe."

Brigitte Botten

Diet culture demonises and shames people in larger bodies, creating a fear of fatness in our society, also known as 'fatphobia.' Fatphobia has encouraged us to assume that people who are overweight are not trying to change their habits. Our society's fear of fat has undoubtedly led people in larger bodies to diet. They have likely tried dieting for years without success, as diets do not work. They are unsustainable and unhealthy, but that's not the message people hear. Instead, they feel like a failure for not 'successfully' dieting.

The rebound effects of dieting that we often don't hear about include gaining more weight, making people more likely to engage in binge eating and develop other disordered eating behaviours. It can also lead to increased chances of nutritional deficiencies, inflammations and fertility concerns, as well as developing a higher risk of heart disease and diabetes. Additionally, feeling stigmatised and ashamed for being in a larger body in our society can cause chronic health problems, such as high blood pressure and increased levels of cortisol.

Yo-yo dieting, formally known as weight cycling, is the starting and stopping of dieting. Weight cycling happens when someone gains weight unintentionally and starts dieting in response, then regains that weight again.

Researchers have associated weight cycling with increased health issues, including high cholesterol, cardiovascular disease, gallbladder disease and mental health issues like depression. An American study by Strohacker, Carpenter and McFarlin called "Consequences of Weight Cycling: An Increase in Disease Risk?" argues that weight cycling increases the risk of developing Type II Diabetes compared to those who maintain a stable weight. They also look into the fact that most people who lose weight will likely not maintain their weight loss long-term. More research needs to occur in this area, as researchers are concerned that weight cycling will become a public health issue.

When I was working in the weight loss industry, I was trying to help people reach their health and wellness goals and, not surprisingly, the main goal that every patient wanted guidance with was weight loss. Now, as an anti-diet intuitive nutritionist and health coach, I would never go back to the weight loss industry. The expectations we put on our patients were unrealistic. Patients were put on super unhealthy, low-calorie diets. Of course, they lost weight quickly because they were not eating, which was unsustainable. There was a common cycle; starve, lose weight, binge eat, gain weight, over-exercise, obsess over food, repeat.

The worst part was that patients thought it was their fault that they had gained the weight back. They blamed themselves, and the weight loss industry let them. After all, it's a money-making industry, and the truth doesn't sell.

The weight loss industry sells the idea that anyone can and should want to lose weight, with biology rarely entering the conversation. Biologically, humans are programmed to eat as if we are still hunters and gatherers. Hundreds of years ago, when we couldn't eat, our inner mechanisms, like our metabolism, would slow down to compensate for the lack of food. When we are not getting enough food, our body retains fat to protect itself and will sacrifice muscle mass. This also happens when we diet. Our hormones send cravings to our brains, telling us to eat foods high in carbohydrates and can provide 'quick energy', like sugar. This is our primal hunger. It makes us lose touch with our fullness, leading to over-eating and panic, telling our brains that we need more food.

It is not the person failing at dieting. Restricted eating sets us up to eat more and punish more. Diets are failing us.

4

Nelly

I am an ex-personal trainer, avid pole dancer, erotic entertainer (erotic dancer, stripper, spicy ballerina, sex worker, whichever you prefer), and frosting-covered snack enthusiast. I started my journey with weight loss like many young, impressionable teenage girls at the beginning of the 21st century by flailing around on my bedroom floor, trying to master the 20-minute fat blaster workout in Cosmo magazine.

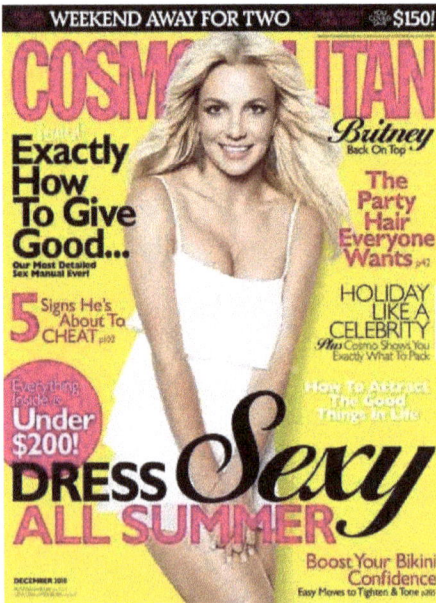

2010 Cosmopolitan Magazine cover.

After becoming a personal trainer and suffering through several eight-week challenges and fad diets, I realised that society's measure of worth was tied primarily to how we look. The pursuit for abs that protruded over hungry stomachs and the obsession with consuming practically no calories was unrelenting. It broke my heart to see so many kind-hearted, incredible women overshadowed by a society that deemed them unworthy of self-love and acceptance because of their weight. I began questioning what the fitness industry called a 'healthy lifestyle' and realised that my happiness, worth and purpose were far more than being young, skinny… and hungry.

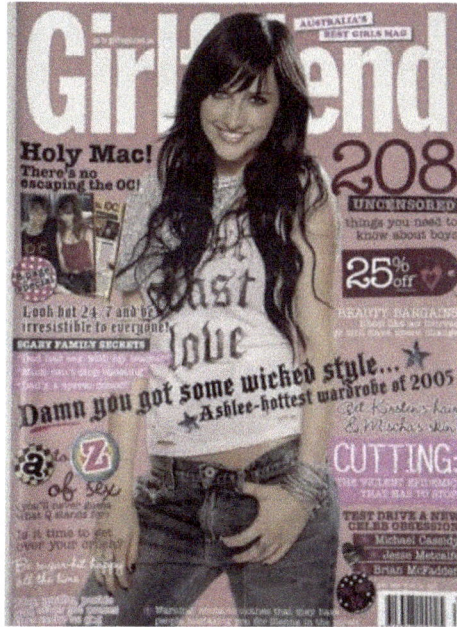

2010 Girlfriend Magazine cover.

One of the most pivotal moments in my life was picking up my first ever Girlfriend Magazine, which my older cousin had gifted me. I didn't know it then, but this would be the moment my worth as a female would change forever. At first, it was as innocent as mimicking the girls' makeup on the cover. It was keeping up with the latest trends draped on emaciated models, and then it was the sinking feeling of realising all the happy, smiling, successful women had one thing in common: they were all thin.

At twenty-one years old, my mother and a close friend seemed surprised to learn that I had a disordered relationship with food. And to be honest, I was too. I felt stupid for being so obsessed with my weight and looks. However, it is no wonder many women spend most of their lives gripped by the obsession with thinness. Why? For so long, the media and publications, like Girlfriend Magazine, have celebrated thinness and its relationship with happiness.

The world praises beauty above all else, so we will feel like we aren't good enough when we don't live up to those standards. What the bombardment of images in the magazines did to me as a teenager was make it very difficult to decide how I felt about my worth to others, particularly men. It appeared that the only women worth loving and praising were the hyper-sexualised and overly thin. Was my stomach flat enough? Did my bra need more padding? Was my skirt short enough, or was it too short?

While I struggled with my body image in my early twenties, I decided to take up a new hobby, pole dancing. I recognise the contradictory nature of the decision to take up a sport in which underwear was the 'uniform' and, professionally, was an industry targeted to entertain men at the expense of a woman's self-worth. Pole dancing and stripping , however, are two very different things that I will discuss later in this chapter.

Attending my first-ever pole dancing class took courage as I felt incredibly nervous about showing up in shorts that were short enough for my butt cheeks to peek out the bottom. On the way to the studio, I nervously pulled my jumper down over my shorts, fearing that my exposed legs were jiggling too much as I walked.

Over the next eight weeks, I felt calm during the classes, which I had never felt before during exercise. Not only was I having fun, but I was also in an environment where aspects of the female body that were typically considered taboo became the norm: pubic hair budding out the sides of booty spanks, cleavage, belly rolls and cellulite proudly taking the spotlight without judgement. Slipping a nipple or a labia while ungraciously straddling the pole in pursuit of achieving a new trick while your classmates cheered you on was a familiar scene in the pole classroom.

As the months went on with pole dancing, I became more in touch with my body than ever before. In the past, I had been told to cover up the parts of my body that made me a woman or the parts that weren't attractive to others; I was now celebrating them shamelessly!

Often, for women to be taken seriously, we feel pressured to abandon our femininity, be ashamed of our sexuality and behave in a certain masculine way. For me, when people learned that I was pole dancing, their reaction was often a raised eyebrow and scrutiny. I would justify my behaviour by responding to their judgement with, "Oh, but I'm not a stripper. Stripping and pole dancing aren't the same thing."

As the years went on, I started to realise that I was not doing the 'sisterhood' any favours by inexplicitly shaming a group of women for having different life choices than me.

Along my journey in the pole dancing industry, it became more and more common for erotic style dancing and pole dancing to integrate. Erotic style dance classes became more popular as many women, including myself, enjoyed feeling sexy without the pressures of society's standards.

One day after an erotic floor class, I overheard my instructor chatting to one of the students about the strip clubs they worked at part-time. I remember thinking, but… you don't seem like strippers. My ignorance of the industry shone through at this moment, but after a breakup at the age of twenty-six, I decided, why not give it a go?

On my first night dancing professionally, I was full of apprehension; what if the girls weren't nice? What if the bosses are mean? What if I'm not good enough? But stepping out onto the stage, all I felt was the freedom I got whenever I danced. Profoundly, I quickly realised that the world does not write the rules on my body; I do.

In my early days of dancing, I cemented a core belief that I will carry for the rest of my life; that I set the boundaries on my body. How my body looks and what I choose to do with it are not indicators of my worth.

Now, I am not saying my line of work is for everyone, but giving women expressive spaces in their lives, as the pole dancing community had done for me, allows us to become confident in our bodies outside the realms of societal expectation, and gives the power back to women to nurture their relationship with their bodies.

All too often, we must have it one way or the other. We either need to hold onto our youth and beauty or relinquish all ties to how we feel about our bodies so that our other attributes can be noticed. But can't we have it all? My truth is, like with everything, it will never be black and white. Our bodies are vessels to carry us through life and are also a part of who we are. We can simultaneously enjoy what our bodies can do and how they look while knowing that there are many other essential and worthy parts of ourselves, regardless of what the world has told us.

5

Nelly: Perspective

My eldest brother's wedding was one of the most pivotal moments in my journey to body acceptance. Months before the big day, I was having a tiff with myself in the changerooms at Myer. I'd been experiencing problems at work and in my relationship that had caused me to stress eat, resulting in my arms looking not as slender as I wished they would in my bridesmaid's dress. I felt disappointed and could only think about how I would look in the wedding photos, angry for 'letting myself go' slightly. I tried to put all these worries behind me on the weekend of the wedding. My boss's nagging requests stayed at the door on Friday afternoon, I side-lined my arguments with my partner that week and postponed any errands until Monday. We'd all been waiting for this day for months.

We spent the morning of the wedding getting hair and makeup done while laughing over champagne and chocolate-coated strawberries with the bride and other bridesmaids. My mother held the hands of her future daughter-in-law with joy-filled tears in her eyes, and I hugged my sister-in-law with excitement after all the months of planning had come together for this one fairytale day. The wedding was filled with warm, long-awaited hugs from extended family I hadn't seen in years, laughing with friends and seeing just how much joy these two special people in my life had created. At the end of the night, my mother, my other brother, and I piled into a taxi with a bottle of champagne and a multitude of desserts from the buffet. It wasn't until a few days after the wedding that I realised something about that day, that it was the happiest day of my life so far, and I didn't once worry about how my arms looked in my dress or how many pieces of cake I ate.

My heart had never felt so full to see how much love I had and how lucky I was to have people that made me feel that way. I know they will always love me, regardless of my body. After this, I realised the answer to moving away from my obsession with my weight was not any diet or exercise plan but rather re-focusing on all the wonderful aspects of my life I already had. When I look back on the years of my misguided pursuit of happiness, I remember fondly not the moments when I was a slave to my eating habits. I don't know what day I hit my most significant weight loss or when I bought my first smaller pair of jeans. I remember the adventures I'd been on, the countries I'd visited and all the laughter I'd shared with friends and family. I felt that the world had tried to make those things seem less important than my weight, but I now know better. My relationship with my body was not fixed completely in a day, but it was a catalyst for me to be able to put the importance of my weight into the perspective of everything else in my life. I began asking myself why it mattered so much, what I felt I was lacking, and what it was that truly brought me peace in life.

Many of us find it hard to accept that our youth and beauty are fleeting. I know the 'peak' of my beauty in societal terms is coming, and soon, my body will begin to change. As this happens, I hope to remember a sobering thought I had after my brother's wedding, *spending a life believing happiness is only reserved for those of a certain size would be a monumental waste of time.*

6

Mary: Disorder

"In all chaos there is a cosmos, in all disorder a secret order."

Carl Jung

As a social worker, I am continuously meeting people who disclose that they are experiencing body image issues and disordered eating, even if that is not the main issue they come to me with. Sometimes, it seems too overwhelming or too big of a problem to handle when I think about how many people this affects. But when I realised this overwhelming feeling was due to a lack of information, I knew I needed more education. Then, I would also be able to give people as much information as possible so that they can make informed choices. To help myself understand more about disordered eating and eating disorders, I met with a brilliant clinical psychologist, Dr Emma Black, whose passion focuses on supporting women in improving their lives. Before she became a clinical psychologist, Dr Black saw firsthand the affects eating disorders had on the people she cared about. She also saw the difference a good practitioner could make in that person's life.

I was so excited she agreed to meet with me. We sat down at a small white table in a boutique cafe filled with indoor plants, handmade gifts and linen clothes for sale, along with a shelf filled with cakes and scones. The café was buzzing with happy customers and busy staff. We were served our coffee and cake and dove into deep interview-style conversation.

Q. What issues do you hear about the most from clients?

A. All of the women who come to see me are unhappy with their bodies, and they all want to be thinner, no matter what size they are. They have all heard unhelpful comments about their bodies from their families, their friends, or peers, encouraging them to lose weight. They are taught to believe that being skinny is essential, and they, therefore, constantly need to be taking steps to become skinny. Their self-worth is linked to the steps they are taking to be skinny.

It is also a desire that most people have to be in control of something in their lives. They can't control all these other things happening but can control their eating. You don't have to feel your feelings if you are binge eating or starving. The vicious cycle is that when you are restricting your eating, you feel like you are in control, and when you binge eat because you are just so hungry, you feel you have lost control. Then, you punish yourself with negative self-talk, and the cycle starts again.

When I start working with someone, there is usually an identity struggle; they often believe they ARE the disorder they have been diagnosed with. So, to challenge that, we explore who the person is.

I honestly forgot I had a coffee in front of me. I drank half of it in two gulps, and then I tried to contribute to the conversation and told Dr Black that I hear the term 'body dysmorphia' a lot these days. I understand it is when you obsess over a flaw or multiple flaws in your appearance; sometimes, the flaws aren't even fundamental.

Q. If you have an eating disorder, does that mean you have body dysmorphia?

A. Not everyone who has an eating disorder has body dysmorphia. They could be living with body dissatisfaction, which is more common in my work.

Body dissatisfaction? I hadn't heard that term before. What started as a few short questions had now snowballed into an hour-long interview. The more questions she answered, the more questions I had.

Q. How many types of eating disorders are there?

A. Many. The DSM (Diagnostic and Statistical Manual) used to only name Anorexia and Bulimia as the most known eating disorders and put all others under Not Otherwise Specified, which were the majority. The DSM has now specified more diagnoses, including binge eating and purging.

Purging, I have learned, is different from Bulimia. With purging, the person typically eats very little before self-induced vomiting. Bulimia, however, is when a person usually binge eats and then focuses their energy on not gaining any weight either by excessive exercising, fasting or vomiting. Any eating disorder is a recognised mental illness and can increase a person's risk of self-harm, unintended death and suicide. (Butterfly Foundation, 2022).

Q. What could be the cause of body image issues and eating disorders for women in Australia?

A. A series of unhelpful behaviours that people undertake to manage and cope with stress while trying to reach an ideal body type. Western culture focuses on a thinner body as an ideal body type. Social and family pressures contribute to this. Women and girls are actively learning that their bodies are not OK just as they are. They believe the criticisms told to them and start taking steps to reach their ideal body. They are taught to diet. Dieting turns into other unhelpful behaviours, including following rules and restrictions, like fasting. Strict rules need to be revised. People naturally rebel when they are being restricted. Tight restrictions always create more problems.

Q. What approach do you use in your work as a Clinical Psychologist?

A. Every practitioner is different, but Clinical Psychologists like me use an evidence-based approach. This means that once there is a diagnosis, we can use specific appropriate therapies. The treatment for someone with Anorexia would be different to the treatment for someone with Bulimia.

There is also an approach called trans-diagnostic intervention, which can be used across different diagnoses. Still, this treatment is specifically tailored to the individual. This approach often includes CBT-E (Cognitive Behavioural Therapy – Enhanced). Also, even though I work within a Medical Model, I know I am engaging with people, not a diagnosis, and people are complicated.

Q. What does recovery look like?

A. Recovery from a Medical Model perspective means a reduction of symptoms. Recovery from a Personal Model perspective means an individual can regain a quality of life and learn to live with the symptoms. It's sometimes not about losing symptoms. Sometimes, it's just about getting to live your life.

A recent systematic review by Wetzler, Hackmann and Peryer (2020) pooled research that examined recovery from people's lived perspectives and what this involved. This review comprised 20 studies, with 351 participants with various eating disorder diagnoses in their history. Several key themes emerged as necessary for recovery:

1. Supportive relationships: Receiving support and encouragement from others and feeling connected to other people. Peer support from people who were in recovery also made a difference.

2. Hope: This is believing that it is possible to recover and have a better future that is not controlled by the eating disorder. This belief can help people push through when the going gets tough.

3. Identity: This is discovering who you are and your interests and

realising that you are not your eating disorder or weight.

4. Meaning and purpose: Identifying why the eating disorder developed. It's also learning that there is more to life than the eating disorder and that there is purpose outside of this.

5. Empowerment: Regaining control over your life rather than having it controlled by the eating disorder.

6. Self-compassion: Learning how to be kind to yourself. This can involve easing the self-criticism, practising self-care, and becoming aware of your needs and emotions and honouring these.

Q. How can we try to prevent or reduce the risk of eating disorders?

A. We need to educate ourselves. Read books! My top recommendations are '8 Keys to Recovery' by Carolyn Costin and Gwen Schubert Grabb and 'Overcoming Binge Eating' by Christopher Fairburn.

Q. What is the most significant thing you have learned through your work?

A. I learned the hard way that you cannot always follow a formula. Eating disorders are complex, and other issues usually accompany them. People cannot follow a narrow path for treatment.

Q. What is the most important message that you want to share?

A. Recovery is possible. If you are living with an eating disorder now and you do not have hope, with the proper support, hope can be developed. An eating disorder is a cycle that you can break. Also, instead of using the extreme labels of 'body negativity' and 'body positivity' that are popular these days, it is more realistic to be 'body neutral.' This means simply accepting our bodies. We can like different parts of our bodies more than other parts. It does not have to be all hate or all love. It's neutral. It's grey.

Our coffee cups were empty, but my head and heart were full. Before our meeting ended, we acknowledged that we both have experience working in the domestic and family violence field. I noticed that the advice I give to supportive friends and family members of those who have experienced domestic and family violence is the same advice Dr Black would give to those whose loved ones are living with an eating disorder; "Don't act like a perpetrator. Don't try to control them or their choices. All you can do is support them and give them information to help them make their own choices."

7

Mary: Shredded

According to the Butterfly Foundation website, around 37% of people in 2022 diagnosed with eating disorders in Australia were male. I think it's important to note that statistics are never perfect, and it's highly likely that the number of males experiencing eating disorders could be even higher.

However, it seems people in general accept the idea of men adopting a more fitness-centric lifestyle; spending a lot more time and energy focused on exercise and restricted eating, without people questioning it. I have always assumed that it is easier for men to achieve the ideal body type because they

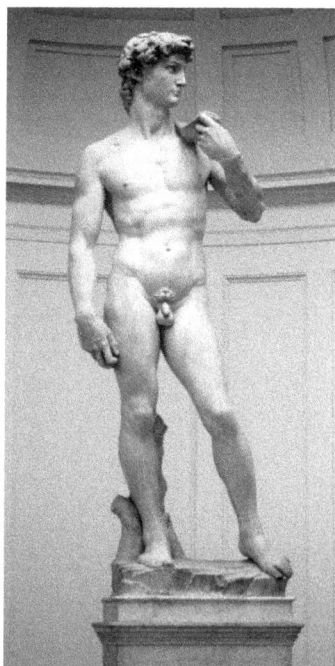

Michelangelo's David, completed in 1504, a famous symbol of independence, strength, youth and beauty.

have higher testosterone, but it takes a lot more than hormones to look like a Greek god. If the level of a man's commitment to exercise and protein intake became extreme or unhealthy, would anybody notice? If he seems confident, is he? If he's shredded, is he enough now?

When writing the first pages of this book, I started following the men's mental health podcast 'Young Blood: Men's Mental Health,' hosted by Callum MacPherson. I came across a discussion in this podcast about fitness, bodybuilding and body image issues for men, so I contacted Callum, who agreed to have a ZOOM video call with me.

Side note: I highly recommend this podcast as each intriguing episode addresses life experiences and perspectives shared vulnerably through the lens of men's mental health.

I asked Callum questions about male perspectives on body image in general, reflecting on his conversations on his podcasts. During our discussion, I sheepishly addressed Callum's appearance, noting that he was well-groomed and noticeably toned. Callum was humble, open and honest when answering questions about himself and sharing his philosophies on male body image.

Callum: *At school, I was always paid out for being skinny, anorexic, a stick. Calling a boy skinny is like calling a girl fat in the way that it goes against the ideal body type. My way of reacting to that was to tease others for being overweight because I could eat whatever I wanted and stay skinny, and they couldn't. With societal changes like women and men being more equal in the workplace, higher divorce rates and so on, the idea of 'men' has become disenfranchised. Men's roles are changing, which can leave young men feeling unsure. Even when I had no idea what I was doing in my life, at least I could focus on my body. I could control that. People respected me for it. It is a very straightforward way of being a 'man', and I can feel surer about myself.*

Callum appeared quite reflective of the contributions fitness and body image have made to his life. On the one hand, it helps with his identity as a man and helps him achieve goals as an individual. On the other hand, societal pressures influence him, like everybody, to compare himself to others.

Callum: *I have been training for over ten years. My fitness and training are my foundations, which enable me to do all the other things that are meaningful to my life. However, I am vain. When I don't get enough sun, I use a tanning lotion. I don't like to have any body hair because it will cover muscle definition. When I go to the beach and feel I am not at my own physical best, I feel self-conscious.*

Callum explained that for him as a man, his fitness and appearance help him feel confident, when necessary, to avoid being the submissive one in a group.

"I know it is very lizard brain," he said.

He described situations where men would gather, mainly in a professional setting but also in social settings and, subconsciously or not, size each other up. They try to figure out who they can trust, who they can respect, who has their shit together and who is in control. Callum clarified that if he is ever lacking in some other area, his appearance will often make up for it, and other men will see him as competent.

I empathised with Callum. As women, we have more access to makeup, hairstyles and clothing to make us look confident and important. Apart from facial hair, a suit and a good skincare routine, men don't have much to work with that mainstream society accepts as the norm. It makes sense. Suppose you see a man who has put effort into sculpting his body a certain way through years of discipline. You may then be more likely to believe that this man would be disciplined enough to achieve challenging goals in the workplace, in sport, in life.

"If it were easy, it would drop in value, and people wouldn't look up to it," Callum explained.

Callum also pointed out that he sees the lies advertised by the fitness industry too. Still, his mindset allows him to see all the benefits of having a fitness lifestyle.

Callum: *Gyms have those posters for 12-week fitness programs with a photo of a shredded professional athlete. Then people get disappointed because they don't look like that after 12 weeks. Try a 12-month program. It's a slow process but more realistic. For me, training also makes me feel sharp. If I train in the morning, I am good to go for the rest of the day. I can be more articulate and more confident. I do get female attention, but most of the positive feedback about my body comes from men. Men hype each other up about their appearance, just like women hype each other up. Fitness can be positive as long as it's not the only thing in your life. I am not my body. But I wouldn't judge someone whose job is centred around their body, like a bodybuilder.*

I have always liked exercising. Who hates endorphins? I exercise in a way I enjoy. If someone told me that exercising was going for a run in a group, there's no way I would do that. Maybe people who say they don't enjoy exercising just haven't found an enjoyable way to exercise that works for them. If you can reach the point where you like exercising or training, your mental health will benefit. You can also enjoy the feeling of working towards something. Still, it's better that you are happy with yourself in the process rather than forbidding yourself to be happy until you reach the desired physical result. Also, improving your physical appearance or level of fitness to prove someone wrong is only going to harm your mental health and wellbeing.

I asked Callum what he thought about the media's influence over body image.

Callum: *It is a well-accepted fact that the media has a monstrous influence over how people think about fitness, health and body image. It's all in good marketing.*

Furthermore, if you put fitness as an interest on your social media profile, you will see an increase in fitness related posts. So, you are shown a false portrayal of 'normal.' I believe that the health and fitness industries are not about health and fitness at all. The model on the protein powder posters is a professional bodybuilder or athlete, not a regular guy who enjoys fitness and protein supplements. There is pressure on men, around how they should look, mainly shown through social media. Images of the ideal body type are thrown in everyone's face. People are being exposed to this at a much younger age because of the accessibility to social media platforms like Snapchat and TikTok, where not just famous people have ideal bodies, but so do 'normal' people.

It is easier to sell the idea of losing weight or gaining muscle quickly. Why wait? Why make a long-term investment in yourself when you are told you can get there in a fraction of the time?

Callum speaks a little further on the fitness industry, mainly bodybuilding, stating that even if someone plays the long game and achieves their goal muscle mass, they spend many years trying to maintain something that will eventually become unmaintainable.

Callum: *Some people say they can gain 10kg of lean muscle annually. That's crazy. If you do everything right, you could gain 1kg of lean muscle a year, which is great progress. When you start training, you feel powerful, and when you start seeing changes, you feel proud, but after a while, that stops, and you try to maintain where you are unless you want to get on the drugs. That's the truth of it but I don't believe the truth sells.*

8

Mary: Shame

At the time of coming up with chapter ideas for this book, the Body Positivity Movement was taking the social media stage by storm. However, I noticed along with the movement came a backlash of criticism, accusing the movement of encouraging people to be unhealthy and fat.

Of course, the solution is not to body shame someone with a thin body, toned body, fat body or anybody. But suppose we realise there can be health within every body type. In that case, the media and the fitness and weight loss industries won't control our choices about our bodies anymore.

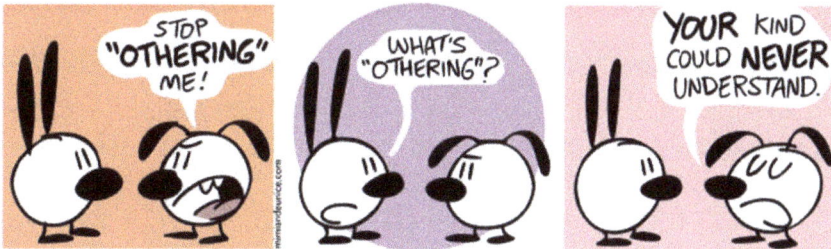

Mimi and Eunice animation by Nina Paley, 2010.

Unfortunately, the painful side to social media is that people with low self-esteem could listen to negative messages delivered by influencers who prioritise getting more views over sharing helpful information, resulting in severely worsening their mental well-being and, subsequently, their physical well-being. Sometimes, the messages we get through the media make people feel like they are not good enough, that they don't belong, or are 'other.'

Humans strive for a sense of belonging. So why do we easily label people as 'other' and make assumptions about them? The answer is not that complicated. We haven't evolved as much as a species in this area. It is simply survival of the fittest. To survive in our tribe, we need to be accepted by the tribe. Anyone who threatens the thoughts and beliefs of the tribe is seen as a threat to its lifestyle. They must be destroyed. So, we shame them. When we lack this social awareness and are too afraid to challenge our beliefs, we end up tearing people down instead of building them up. Attacking someone's appearance is easy. It also ensures that the pack stays tight-knit and at an ideal amount with a manageable number of problems. They are more likely to survive the sabre tooth tigers. But more commonly than not, people choose to challenge their caveman brains and not be threatened by those who look different from what they are used to. We are continuously busting the status-quo wide open and exposing it to different and exciting ways of living, which are much less easily controlled.

On the other end of the spectrum, I have seen the society I live in put people who appear different, people who would rarely take the media spotlight, like fat people, front and centre. But this was not to empower them. No. It was to judge, shame and be entertained by them. The example I am thinking of is a show that sensationalised obesity and gave contestants the same attention they would provide people with deformities, displayed as circus freaks in the 19th century. Thankfully, the TV show 'The Biggest Loser' is no longer airing on Australian television. The name in itself is deliberately derogatory. This reality TV show ran for 10 seasons in Australia and 18 seasons in America . It was finally cancelled after medical reports of starvation tactics and whispers of rigged weigh-ins were leaked to the public. Not to mention the bullying rumours. It surprises me how long this show was allowed to run, seeing as so many contestants both in the American and Australian series gained most of their weight back after their season ended.

Not only do extreme exercise and dieting negatively affect our metabolism, but lapsing back to old eating habits afterwards is almost guaranteed. Because all the life problems have not gone away, and new coping strategies have not been learned. It's like sending someone to an intense rehab program and then sending them back out into the world with no support whatsoever. What if they lapse? Well, shame on them; they failed! They failed because they still had the same life problems they had before they entered rehabilitation.

We have been sold the idea that extreme exercise and dieting will get someone to lose weight very quickly. Still, we forget that the weight will be gained back the moment we stop torturing ourselves with starvation, obsession over calories and intense workout routines. After all that effort, the only thing that is likely to be maintained is severe mental health issues and plummeting self-esteem.

For years, we were entertained by a show that celebrated the thinnest, cough; I mean the fittest person of the week by placing them on top of a large pedestal in the form of an industrial scale in front of a studio audience. If they lost the most weight at the end of the season, they were showered with gold streamers while the audience chanted and cheered for them. They did it! They lost the weight! Society accepts them!

Now, some may argue with me that I am encouraging obesity and, therefore, the health risks that come with it. Of course, I am not encouraging people to put their health at risk. Rather, we should not judge other people because of their weight and assume the right to decide they have less value.

The journey of nurturing our physical and mental health is not reserved for those labelled as obese, just as much as it is not reserved for professional athletes. The journey of meeting our nutritional needs to reduce the risk of disease, infection, and premature death while increasing our levels of happy hormones, energy and enjoyment of movement, sex and sleep is a life-long commitment. It is everyone's journey, and shame has no place in it.

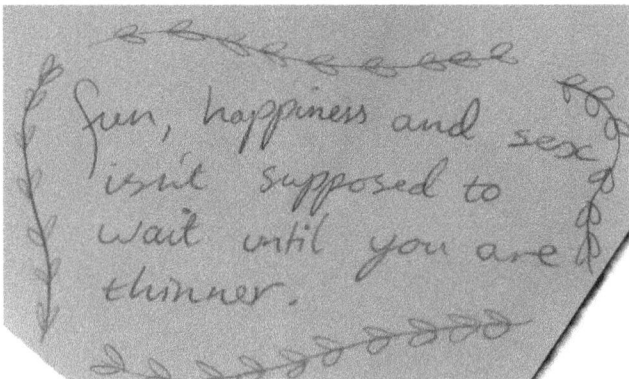

Pearson's note at the back of a notebook, June 2023.

9

Mary: Where to from here?

The media, the fitness industry and the weight loss industry, have been the perpetrators of body image issues for what feels like millennia. But we must also take responsibility for the part we play. How often do we say we must be 'good' with so much conviction when refusing food? How much less do we celebrate people who don't fit the eating behaviours or beauty standards we think they should? How deeply do we believe we are not good enough, and how do these thoughts influence those we may be setting an example for? If we want to contribute to real change, we can. We can reduce the number of lives lost each year due to eating disorders, which surpasses the number of road accident mortalities (Butterfly Foundation, 2022). Arming ourselves with knowledge and connecting with support is the way forward.

Professionally, I have always felt some degree of self-doubt about not having enough in common with people in order to connect with them, especially if they look, sound or act differently to me. This is imposter syndrome at its finest. In the same way, I questioned if people could relate to this book if they weren't like the people writing it. Wrong again. We don't have to have suffered through what others have to be able to relate to them. If I did, I would be one immensely traumatised social worker. Not that there isn't still time for that!

It is our empathy and curiosity that makes us connect with people, a story, or a book. Therefore, it has been decided that this book's target demographic is anyone who finds it attractive.

That being said, addressing two demographics who may want to pursue this area further after they turn the last page is necessary.

Those who connect personally with the stories in this book and struggle with their relationship with their body, food and fitness, are Group A. Those who are helplessly watching a loved one experiencing this struggle, are Group B. Here are my recommendations for each group to consider.

Disclaimer: The recommendations that follow are not specific to any one person's situation and are in no way medical advice. I am sharing insights from a social worker's perspective, influenced by multidisciplinary professional experiences that have helped me personally and professionally.

Group A

Step One: Educate yourself as much as possible.

Understand the science behind your thoughts, feelings and behaviours. There are plenty of books, articles, and videos you can use to arm yourself with enough knowledge to analyse your situation. Externalising your problems helps to understand them better. It's worth mentioning that proper self-help includes challenging your own bias or perspective, especially if the perspective you already have is causing you suffering. Be open to learning about different and evidence-based perspectives.

I recommend the Australian Centre for Eating Behaviour and the Butterfly Foundation, two Australian organisations that provide up-to-date information about body image and our relationships with food, including eating disorders.

Step Two: Understand your biases.

We all have beliefs, judgments, and stereotypes we accept as truth because we grew up hearing them and never challenging them. Usually, they can be harsh like, 'fat people are lazy, thinner people are happy, if I can't do this I'm a failure, no one will love me while I look like this, other people have it worse, this isn't even a real problem.'

You are not alone if these opposing narratives pass through your mind. It is essential to notice when the thoughts are happening and try to question them.

Where did these thoughts come from?

Does anyone else in your life encourage these thoughts?

Are they facts or assumptions?

This skill takes a lot of practice and sometimes talking to a counsellor or psychologist will help. Right now, these unhelpful beliefs might be standing in the way of the life you want. It's easy to accept these beliefs as truth, as humans are predisposed to accept negative statements about themselves over positive ones. The trick is to accept them as simply thoughts and not as a part of your identity. Your identity is so much more colourful than these self-punishing thoughts. The long-term effects of facing your truths will be well worth the effort.

Step Three: Making a real change.

Ask yourself how close you are to making a fundamental change in your life. Then, try your best to answer. You can do this by knowing what stage of change you are in.

The Stages of Change model was created in the 1980s to help researchers understand human behaviour around smoking (Prochaska & DiClemente, 1994). Today, it is used by mental health professionals all over the place to explore any behavioural change and how humans choose or not choose to do it.

There are five main stages:

1. Pre-contemplation (having no intention of changing a behaviour),

2. Contemplation (being aware that a problem exists, gaining information

but not committing to change),

3. Preparation (committing to taking actions to change a behaviour),

4. Action (physically making efforts to change a behaviour, like a social experiment but on yourself) and,

5. Maintenance (replacing the old behaviour with new behaviours and using strategies to sustain this in your everyday life).

This model acknowledges that people often lapse into unhelpful or destructive behaviours, needing to start the stages again. The word 'lapse' is used rather than 'relapse' because people don't start from the beginning, they start the stages again with new knowledge and experiences; therefore, each time is different. The model says that people make mistakes, but there are always steps to help us try again depending on how dedicated we are to getting the life we want.

Suppose you are in the contemplation, preparation or action phase. In that case, organisations like the ones I mentioned in step one is an excellent place to start looking for a trained professional to talk to. I always feel more comfortable sharing my story and learning new things face-to-face with someone who knows their shit. There is also the option of talking to your GP and asking for a mental health care plan to get a referral for a psychologist or counsellor in your area at a subsidised or no cost.

Now, if you are one of those rarely-thanked, soldiering-on souls who are watching a loved one struggle with their body, their food and their health, my steps follow the same pattern but with slight tweaks.

Group B

Step One: Educate yourself as much as possible.

If you are anything like me, you have already done this. You are now struggling because no matter what you do, the person you care about is unwilling to listen. Take it from a social worker: no one wants to be told what to do. The individual is the expert in themselves. If they are in the pre-contemplation phase, often we are limited to simply telling them that we are concerned about them because we have noticed certain behaviours, assuring them that we are a safe place to come to when they are ready to talk about it. Sometimes, this honest conversation is powerful enough to show the person how serious the situation is, and they may open up. Equally as possible, they might come across as highly reassuring, delivering a confident lie telling you that everything is fine. Please don't take this personally. Lying or denial about any harm towards one's self is very common. You can sit a little longer in awkward, uncomfortable energy and, as caring as possible, reassure them that you are still concerned and will be ready to listen when they are prepared to talk.

Step Two: Know what your biases are, too.

You might be very close to this person, so you are interested in them and their wellbeing. But it is important to understand that your goals and dreams for them might be very different from what they want. It's important to reflect on what you want for them and why. Where does it come from? It might be hard for them to be completely honest with you because they will likely fear letting you down, upsetting you, or being judged. This is normal. In the initial stages of talking to this person about your concerns, try not to influence them to make the changes you want them to make to their behaviour; they'll see right through that. Ask them what they need from you. If it is to do nothing and you feel you simply cannot do nothing, you can negotiate. You can also take a break and talk again a few days later. Remember that the idea here is not to judge but to let them know that you accept them whilst still having your concerns. Unfortunately, caring about someone opens us up to more possibilities for pain. That's the deal, I'm afraid. So, if you are experiencing significant emotional pain worrying about this person, it just means you care so damn much, which is usually a good thing.

Step Three: Are you in front, beside or behind?

One of my first social work lecturers started a class by saying, "Know where you stand with your client! Are you in front, beside or behind?"

My ears pricked up, motivating me to write down every word.

"If you are in front, this must mean that their house is on fire (meaning they are in a crisis which is threatening their life) and they need immediate assistance. Most people are unable to make decisions because of the crisis they are in. Therefore, you are justified to pull them out of the fire.

If you are beside them, they have accepted your support but are not yet ready to go on the journey alone, so you stay close for reassurance. You check in with them and discuss the next steps together. You make plans together, call support services together, make appointments together, and so on. They take the initiative with all decisions and actions.

If you are behind them, you are simply cheering them on. You can still check in with them but not as often, and you can encourage them to continue their progress to get closer to the life they want."

The lecturer continued, "Your position will change depending on where the person is. When and where you want them to be will likely be very different to where they actually are. Meet them where they are and go at their pace. If they want you beside them, you cannot stand before them. If you are burning out and feel overconcerned about this person, even more concerned than they are, look at where you are standing about them. If you are not taking care of yourself, how do you expect to meet them where they are when they are ready to accept your support?"

These powerful words are inspired by a well-known social work theory I have long forgotten the name of. Still, they are relevant enough for me to repeat them here. It is also essential for you to seek support from a medical professional, psychologist or counsellor yourself. They will likely have strategies you can use to communicate with the person you are concerned about or help with coping when feeling unable to fix the problem. I guess that's what it is: coping, most of the time.

10
Mary: Reality

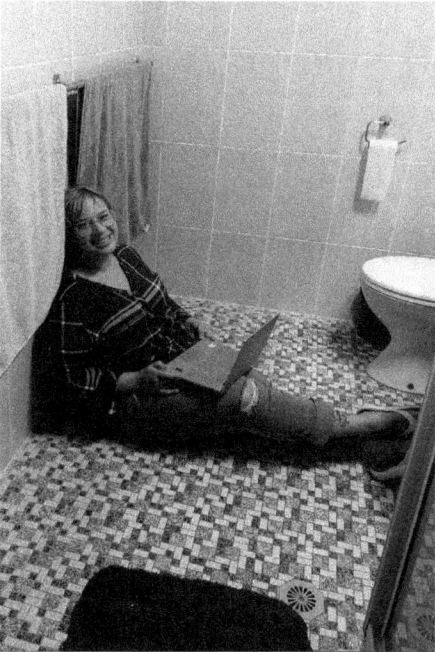

Author, Mary Pearson, writing her final pages of 'Weighed Down' on the bathroom floor.

I wanted to write a poetic finish to this book and wrap all the catchy phrases and facts in a neat bow. But that isn't realistic. What is realistic is that right now I am sitting on my bathroom floor, waiting until my bowels make me dash to the toilet. I am trialling some iron tablets that my doctor says are supposed to help me. But it's been over two months, and I feel no better, just cramped. They told me to take vitamin C tablets or drink orange juice, but that hasn't helped either. Low iron is common for women, but I decided to give the tablets a go instead of increasing my spinach, beans, and meat intake any further. But my gut hurts too much, and I don't think I'll be taking these tablets much longer.

I feel this story is relevant because my GP also prescribed me cholesterol medication on the same day. After seeing the results of my blood test, she said my cholesterol was a tiny bit high, which is strange for a woman who just turned thirty. She told me I had three options:

1. Adjust my diet to have less fried food and dairy.

2. Get a referral to a nutritionist to make a diet plan.

3. Be prescribed cholesterol medication.

I insisted that I am capable of reducing fried food and dairy on my own, though talking about it that way made me feel pretty shitty for demonising foods that I not only enjoy but don't even consume weekly.

I said to her, "Maybe I'm just chubby," with a shrug and a chuckle.

The doctor prescribed me the medication anyway to 'nip it in the bud,' and hopefully, the number on the screen will go down after my next blood test.

A month later, I needed a refill of the cholesterol medication, but I couldn't find my script. I made a quick appointment with whichever GP was available at the same clinic. This time, it was not my regular GP, a polite and well-spoken woman in her early thirties, but a man in his late fifties with the disposition of someone sick of talking to idiots all day.

He looked at my file and, after a few seconds, started to explain to me that my regular GP had made a mistake and my cholesterol levels were acceptable. I was relieved to hear that.

Then, unnecessarily, he explained how to reduce cholesterol levels; "Just have a good diet and exercise. It's easy. Eat vegetables and meat, less dairy and NO JUNK FOOD."

I smiled at him. I couldn't help it. I was amused and disappointed. I wanted to say, "Oh perfect, I was hoping to feel patronised today. Thanks for asking me about all the good things I do for my body. Too bad my cholesterol is just fine, as you said." But instead, I thanked him and left as swiftly as possible.

When I heard the doctor talk in terms of 'no to this food' and 'yes to that food,' I felt sad for other patients who are encouraged to view food as good and bad, as well as being told that losing weight is an easy thing to do, so if you can't there must be something wrong with you. But as the doctor said to me before he passed on advice that was not relevant, I am healthy. I decided to take that information and focus on enjoying being healthy.

I know my body will change throughout my life. I will never look like I did when I was twenty-one and I'll never again have the same metabolism I did when I was sixteen. I might have a baby one day, and my body will change. One day, I will go through menopause, and my body will change again. I will continue to judge some parts and love other parts, and I will continue to love food.

Damn, I do love food. It gives me nutrition and comfort. It is so many things other than something to eat. Food is a Nonna passing down family recipes. It's eating satay skewers on the streets of Jogjakarta and drinking hot tea while admiring Tasmanian snow-capped mountains. It's birthday cakes, anniversary chocolates and tomato soup when I'm sick. Food is medicine. It's adding chia seeds to my yogurt for more fibre and milo to my ice cream for more flavour. When we are kinder to ourselves and decide to enjoy life a little more, we can open our minds to all the beautiful foods out there. Some will give us energy, and others will make us sleepy. Without feeling ill, I can't eat a whole packet of sour worm lollies anymore, but I still love sour worms.

The inconvenient truth is that you will be told that you are not enough throughout your life. The fitness industry, the weight loss industry, the media, and even some closer to home have no problem trying to convince us of that. If the voices around us start to quiet down, a lot of the time, the voices in our minds will pick up the slack and continue telling us that we are not enough. But what if you are? What if I had a crystal ball and told you that the way your body is now is the best it will be? What if I told you to throw out that old outfit from five years ago that doesn't fit you, because this is the closest you will ever get to your ideal size? Would you live a little differently? Would you live a little more?

My reality is that food is essential for me to enjoy life. I need to understand nutrition to thrive, but that does not mean demonising any food to praise others. My reality is that health includes physical movement in an activity I enjoy, nurturing social and spiritual connections and being kind to my body and mind. They are doing the best they can.

We will always care about our appearance. It is in our biology. Presenting ourselves in ways that society deems attractive helps us thrive. Obstacles are removed, romantic offers are multiplied, and suspicions towards us of unsavoury behaviour are lessoned. This makes sense. But, when it comes to our bodies, should we live in the constant pursuit of approval? Should we watch hundreds of videos of unqualified people telling us to stop eating this and eat more of that? Should every woman strive to be slim and every man strive to be an upside-down triangle?

Or do we pursue a holistic understanding of health, our bodies and our minds and have honest conversations about how to nurture these to experience the most out of our lives?

The reality is… we get one body for this life. It's our job to appreciate it, protect it and care for it as if it were someone we were responsible for, because we are.

Acknowledgements

The world is better when people stand up against a status quo that is hurting us as individuals and as a society.

Thank you to Dr Emma Black for sharing your enlightening knowledge and for your dedication to women's wellbeing.

Thank you to Callum MacPherson for your valuable contribution and for all you do for men's mental health.

References

Beck, J., Beck, A. 2020. Cognitive Behaviour Therapy: Basics and Beyond. The Guilford Press.

Butterfly Foundation. 2022. Eating Disorders: who does it affect? butterfly.org. au

Mackintosh, G. 2016. Weight Management Psychology. Facebook.

Prochaska, J., DiClemente, C. 1994. Changing the Self: Philosophies, Techniques and Experiences. State University of New York Press.

Strohacker, K., Carpenter, K. and McFarlin, B. 2009. Consequences of Weight Cycling: An Increase in Disease Risk? National Library of Medicine.

Wetzler, S., Hackmann, C. and Peryer. 2020. A framework to conceptualize personal recovery from eating disorders: A systematic review and qualitative meta-synthesis of perspectives from individuals with lived experience. Wiley Periodicals, Inc.

About the Author
Mary Pearson

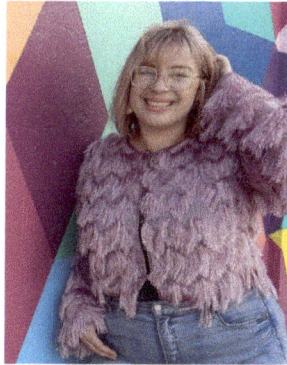

Mary Pearson graduated from Deakin University with a Bachelor's Degree in Social Work with Distinction and a Diploma in Indonesian Language and Culture.

She was a finalist nominee for Queensland's Young Achiever of the Year Award for her work and volunteering efforts for victim-survivors of abuse and is a passionate public speaker. She has also been nominated for Best Aunty, displayed proudly on the front of her fridge.

Today, Mary continues her social work career in North Queensland, specialising in domestic violence but finding herself more frequently in the field of mental health, connecting with people from numerous cultural, age and ability demographics.

Outside of her career, Mary often travels to Indonesia to connect with friends she has met through travel and study opportunities. She visits schools and universities of close friends to share stories of Australian life and history and learns of the tremendous milestones young people are achieving for Indonesia's health and education through activism, from the small streets of Jogjakarta to the universities of Banda Aceh.

On a more personal level, Mary loves the performing arts, especially comedy and theatre; a passion she shares with her parents. Being backstage or waiting in the wings with her siblings for her queue was normal throughout her youth.

She grew up in a small country town in western Victoria with her parents and four siblings. On the weekends, she loved riding the horses owned by a family up the road or swimming in the local river across town. Her fondest memories are of helping her mother in the kitchen by completing the task of scraping the bowl of cake mix and reading the newspaper to her father, which included circling the big words and then looking them up in the dictionary.

"Why try to fit in when you were born to stand out?" Her mother would say, encouraging self-confidence.

"It's never about the right answer; it's about the right question." Her father would say, nurturing Mary's curious and adventurous young mind.

Mary always wanted to be a writer but, like many who have such a dream, was often faced with such self-doubt that she couldn't write anything she liked well enough to show to a publisher. Then, in 2020, at the height of COVID-19, Mary wrote her first children's book for her nephews, 'Shoby Raptor and the Heavy Coat.' The short story is about how feelings are collected throughout the day and may make us feel heavy and worn out, but this is often relieved when we share our feelings with others. After the book was finally published, Mary was motivated to continue writing about what mattered to her.

After hearing a compounding number of stories about people's obsessions with dieting and losing weight and the lies of the fitness and weight loss industries, Mary began to question her own experiences with food and body image and started writing them down. Why did comments about her weight upset her? Why did she feel frustrated when she saw a person at work start diet after diet whilst displaying the most unauthentic smile, trying to reassure others that everything was ok? Why was a mouthful of donuts her go-to option for calming down when overwhelmed by an exam, a job, or a breakup?

Through the underrated art of conversation, she connected with those more well-versed in the weight loss and fitness industries. With her desk covered in yellow sticky notes, Mary finally broached the idea of a short book and shared her thoughts with two dear friends and fellow questioners.

Other titles by Mary Pearson:

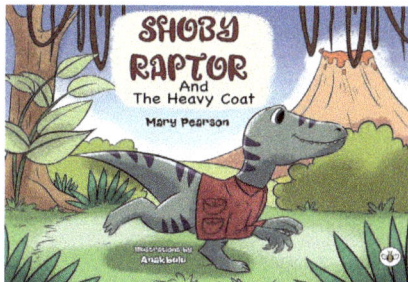

https://olympiapublishers.com/book/shoby-raptor-and-the-heavy-coat

About the Author
Brigitte Botten

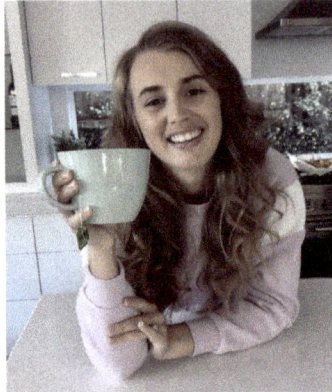

Brigitte fully lives up to her business' name and embraces life. Whether it be while she is travelling abroad or just going for a walk along the beach near her house, whether it's singing at the top of her lungs whilst out dancing to live music or singing in the kitchen whilst creating something delicious, whether it's making new friends (a skill that comes more easily to children) or spending quality time at home with family, Brigitte puts her all into everything.

She grew up in quite a large family with twelve siblings, and it wasn't the picture of your classic Aussie family household. With a bit of money and very little food, Brigitte had to improvise her meals and snacks with whatever they had in the pantry. Pasta with butter and soy sauce, dry Weetbix with peanut butter, tomato sauce and butter sandwiches, to name a few exciting combinations. Now and then, she still craves pasta, butter, and soy sauce for childhood nostalgia.

Brigitte completed her Bachelor in Nutrition at Deakin University in Geelong, where she met Mary, with whom she has now been friends for over a decade.

Soon after finishing university, she moved to America with her partner. Her first job as a nutritional counsellor was at a wellness clinic in Philadelphia. Though she enjoyed establishing relationships with her clients and supporting them in their health journey, she could see first-hand the struggle her clients had when trying to lose the weight they so desperately wanted gone, which got her questioning the health effects of dieting.

She decided to steer her further education away from weight management counselling to a more holistic approach to health and wellness. She completed an Intuitive Eating course under the supervision of the cofounder of Intuitive Eating Pros, Evelyn Tribole and became a Certified Intuitive Eating Counsellor. She also completed an Advanced Certificate in Nutrition and Health Coach at Well College Global to support her new holistic approach. What sat well with Brigitte was understanding that intuitive eating is an integrated mind and body eating style that honours each person's preferences and needs while promoting a healthy attitude towards food and body image.

With these skills and knowledge, Embrace and Nourish was born, and continues with Brigitte at the helm as founder, entrepreneur and intuitive eating nutritionist and health coach.

About the Author
Nelly Rose

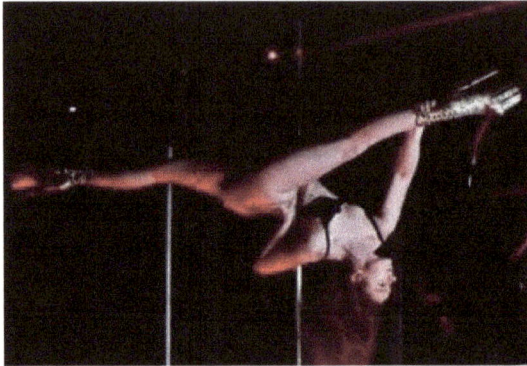

Nelly's career has involved becoming an expert in changing careers. Each time in a different city or country and with different outlooks on life.

After completing her first year of a Bachelor of Arts in Professional and Creative Writing, she decided to switch gears, pursue her passion for horse riding, and study for a Diploma in Horse Business Management. For the years to follow, she spent most of her time around the Victorian, South Australian border riding racehorses at 4 am or taking trail riding groups along the Great Ocean Road.

Having itchy feet, she then moved to Brisbane. She became a personal trainer for her next chapter in life, where she worked mainly with women in group fitness.

Nelly says her views on body image have been on as much of a roller coaster as her career. Having had issues with disordered eating and exercise addiction in her early twenties, it is a topic close to her heart. She went into a personal trainer position, having her obsession with body image disguised as a passion for health and fitness, and it didn't take long to realise this was not an uncommon facade in the fitness industry. She began to understand that her issues and those of her clients ran more profound and complicated than she or the industry was qualified to handle. It filled her with a defeated sadness to see some of her client's self-worth be overshadowed by the societal pressure to be thin. After reflecting on how she saw her body and self-worth, Nelly decided to end her career in the fitness industry until she better understood this relationship.

Her quest for answers found revelation in the seemingly unlikely setting of a change room in New Zealand, in the first strip club she worked at where, she admits sheepishly that up until that moment, she'd never actually seen what naked women's bodies looked like in person. Nelly attributes her time as an erotic dancer to having positively impacted her views of female body diversity, her understanding of bodily boundaries, her female sexual expression and her improved relationships with her fellow female peers.

Today, Nelly resides in Brisbane with her partner and family and travels to various clubs in Australia and New Zealand for erotic dancing. She has a knack for anything creative, with an accolade here or there spread out across her twenties: a few published articles for equine magazines, a national-level pole dancing competition and when she gets the time to sit down, some coloured pencil sketches for her friends.

Nelly has been childhood friends with Mary in their small hometown and has many fond memories with Brigitte during their time at university.

From the Publisher

'Weighed Down' is a captivating explanation of the intricate dance between social beauty norms, self-perception and the pursuit of health. Mary Pearson, along with co-authors Brigitte Botten and Nelly Rose, masterfully explore the impact of our internal dialogues, blending personal anecdotes with researched insights to create an empowering narrative.

As readers embark on this transformative journey, they are encouraged to challenge societal norms and embrace a more accepting and diverse definition of beauty in a world inundated with conflicting messages about appearance and well-being.

'Weighed Down' is a must-read for those seeking to break free from the constraints of judgment and embark on a journey toward embracing the beauty within themselves and others.

Working with Mary on her journey to authorship has been an absolute privilege. I wish her all the best in her endeavours and look forward to more from her and co-authors Brigitte Botten and Nelly Rose.

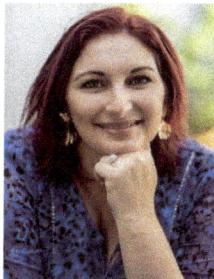

Crystal Leonardi, Bowerbird Publishing
Julatten, Queensland, Australia
www.crystalleonardi.com